ALL ABOUT
HIATUS HERNIA
AND ITS
TREATMENT
WITHOUT DRUGS

ALL ABOUT
HIATUS HERNIA
AND ITS
TREATMENT
WITHOUT DRUGS

By David Potterton ND, MRN, MNIMH
Consultant Medical Herbalist and
Registered Naturopath

foulsham

LONDON • NEW YORK • TORONTO • SYDNEY

foulsham

The Publishing House

Bennetts Close, Cippenham, Berkshire, SL1 5AP

ISBN 0-572-02164-X

Phototypeset in Great Britain by Typesetting Solutions, Slough, Berks
Printed in Great Britain by St. Edmundsbury Press, Bury St Edmunds.

Contents

Preface

Hiatus hernia is a painful and debilitating disease affecting the digestive system. It was rare 60 years ago and, according to medical researchers, is still rare in those parts of the world where people keep to their traditional diets.

In so-called under-developed countries fewer than one person in a hundred has hiatus hernia.

Compare this with Britain and other Western countries where it is estimated that the condition is present to some degree in three out of every ten people under the age of sixty-five.

In those over sixty-five, the incidence rises alarmingly so that seven out of every ten people are affected.

This makes it a disease of major proportions in the UK — one that eats into health service resources, both medical and surgical, yet, in reality, it is a condition that could so easily be prevented.

Medical herbalists and naturopaths are fully qualified to treat hiatus hernia and, if a proper health regimen can be instituted in the early stages, there is every chance that the condition can be reduced or corrected. In advanced cases surgery to repair the hernia may become necessary.

The aim of this book is to describe hiatus hernia syndrome to those who have been properly diagnosed as having the condition and to suggest how natural methods, including herbal and naturopathic treatment may help.

Many of the recommendations given in this book can be undertaken at home and will provide a sound starting point towards recovery.

Of course, success with natural methods depends on self-motivation on the part of the sufferer as it usually means a change in lifestyle.

However, it is always wise to have, if possible, the personal advice and encouragement of a qualified practitioner to help you along the way.

The natural approach does not rely on pharmaceutical drugs for success, but adopts a comprehensive plan of attack to include: attention to diet, control of body-weight, exercises, postural re-education, breathing exercises and advice on lifting heavy objects.

Herbal medicines are prescribed to enhance the healing process, and to relieve symptoms. Vitamin and mineral supplements are also recommended to help build up the general health.

It is not often the case that hiatus hernia is the sole health problem being experienced by the individual. Usually there are associated conditions which also require attention — hence the need for a holistic approach and a reason for referring to hiatus hernia as a syndrome.

Words of Caution

Herbal medicines are generally safe, but they are not without contraindications. Therefore:

1 Never take any herbal medication during pregnancy without advice from a qualified practitioner.

2 Do not treat babies and young children, or the very elderly, without obtaining professional advice as dosages are much more critical.

3 Do not take herbal medicines if you are also taking medicines from your own doctor, as the two may interact. Do not stop taking medicines prescribed by a doctor without advice.

4 Do not self treat if you are suffering from a liver condition or heart disease.

5 Always use herbs from reputable suppliers, but preferably from a medical herbalist. Do not gather medicinal plants from the wild.

Note: Because it is recognised that there are contra-indications and that individuals may react differently to herbal remedies, the author and publishers emphasise that they cannot be held liable for any adverse effects caused by self-treatment with any of the remedies mentioned in this book. Self-treatment must be undertaken according to the individual's own judgement.

Chapter 1

What is Hiatus Hernia?

Although hiatus hernia is a very common defect of the gastrointestinal system, most people will not have heard of it until it is diagnosed by a hospital consultant.

They may have suffered from digestive disturbances for years without realising that a hernia was the real cause of their problem.

However, the mere presence of a hiatus hernia may not be associated with any symptoms at all. It may be diagnosed during a routine screening for another condition and the individual may never have been aware of it.

Usually, it is only when severe digestive symptoms, including chest pains, are being experienced, that people are referred to hospital for further investigation.

The disease occurs more often in the Western world than in under-developed countries and more often in women than in men. It is also more frequent in women who are over-weight. But it can strike anyone at any age.

So exactly what is a hiatus hernia? To put it simply, part of the stomach wall protrudes, or ruptures, through an opening in the diaphragm, the muscle involved in breathing.

Normally, this opening is regulated by a ring of muscular tissue, which acts as a sphincter.

Every time we swallow food the sphincter relaxes and opens, allowing the food to drop into the stomach. It promptly closes again to prevent the food or acid in the stomach from regurgitating back into the throat.

In hiatus hernia the sphincter is unable to work correctly and it is this that is at the root of the digestive symptoms.

One of the main things that a sufferer may complain of is heartburn. This is due to stomach acid leaking through the sphincter and literally burning the oesophagus, or gullet, which, unlike the stomach, has no protection from contact with the acid.

The symptoms tend to come on more when the person bends down to pick up something off the floor, or when they are lying down.

This can be extremely distressing because it means that the pain will often come on at night when the person goes to bed.

When they are lying down the acid can run from the stomach through the sphincter much more easily, causing an unpleasant pain.

It may be that it has been some time since the last meal and, therefore, to feel a pain in the centre of the chest in the middle of the night gives rise to fears of heart disease.

The pain can be cramping, like angina, and may radiate to the neck and arms. Sometimes there are palpitations or heart flutterings.

Some patients worry that they may have stomach cancer because they suffer distension on eating a meal, or they may be sick or discover blood in the stools.

With such severe symptoms most people will see their doctors as soon as possible.

In the milder cases they may be told there is nothing wrong with them, or that they simply have indigestion.

As herbal medicine is particularly good at clearing up

digestive symptoms, medical herbalists tend to see a large number of cases where hiatus hernia has been overlooked.

A busy GP often has little time to go thoroughly into what appears to be a mild digestive disturbance, and is apt to prescribe only a simple antacid treatment, which may indeed, give some relief from the symptoms, but does not remove the underlying cause.

The qualified medical herbalist, or naturopath, will be able to give adequate time to questioning an anxious patient about recurring symptoms and is likely to arrive quickly at an accurate clinical diagnosis.

The treatment, as outlined in this book, will also be holistic and tailored to the individual, rather than being drug-orientated.

Chapter 2

Sliders and Rollers

Sufferers from hiatus hernia can be divided into two groups — the "sliders" and "rollers". I have described hiatus hernia briefly in Chapter one, but to understand it better we need to go into a little more detail.

The sliding hiatus hernia is the more common. What happens is that a part of the stomach, with the sphincter muscle, slides upwards into the chest. A predisposing reason for this is that the oesophagus is shorter in length, possibly since birth, or because it has been burned by acid from the stomach over a period of time.

The sphincter muscle is often operating inefficiently so that inflammatory symptoms, including heartburn, pain, wind, blood-streaked vomiting, and sometimes difficulty in swallowing, may arise.

In severe cases the oesophagus becomes ulcerated and swollen and a blockage may occur.

An individual who has a short oesophagus may only ever complain of indigestion, but many also suffer inflammatory symptoms and pain after eating. They can usually achieve relief from their symptoms by getting into a certain position.

The symptoms experienced by the "rollers" are due to part of the stomach rolling through the opening at the diaphragm, although the sphincter itself operates normally and remains in its proper place below the diaphragm.

A rolling hernia can be triggered by injury, obesity, a chronic cough, or a twisted spine. Many of the spinal cases are diagnosed by osteopathic practitioners.

Because the sphincter is not affected, acid-related symptoms are not the main complaints. Patients are more likely to complain of flatulence, pain or discomfort in the middle of the chest and difficulty in swallowing. A watch has to be kept for anaemia as there may be slight but frequent internal bleeding.

HIATUS HERNIA IN BABIES

Babies are sometimes born with a hiatus hernia. In earlier times it was thought that hiatus hernia in adults was just a development of the infant, or congenital form. Statistics have proved otherwise. Because there are many more cases of hiatus hernia in adults than in children this alerted researchers to look for other causes.

In babies suspicion of hiatus hernia is aroused if there is failure to thrive, particularly if the baby vomits after feeds.

As in adults a barium meal helps to diagnose the condition. However, the treatment of babies suffering from hiatus hernia is very specific, and outside the scope of this book.

Chapter 3

Understanding Heartburn

Heartburn is often the main symptom in the sliding type of hiatus hernia.

There is a burning sensation or discomfort in the middle of the chest and up to the throat.

The discomfort is due to food in the stomach being regurgitated into the lower end of the oesophagus. Regurgitation itself does not normally cause symptoms, so the discomfort is most likely to arise when there is also inflammation present in the oesophagus. This inflammation is known as oesophagitis.

If the inflammation is severe there may also be pain due to oesophageal spasm (see Achalasia).

Regurgitation of food is most likely to occur after meals, on changing one's posture such as by bending to pick up something, or when lying flat in bed at night.

Quite commonly, the sufferer also complains of regurgitation of a sour, bitter fluid.

Heartburn alone is not necessarily a sign of hiatus hernia as it can also occur in pregnancy and in people who are overweight — especially after a large meal.

It is also frequent in diseases of the gall bladder and in people with duodenal ulcer when there is excessive acid in the stomach.

Heartburn in pregnancy is likely, of course, to be much worse if the woman also has a hiatus hernia. This is because there is a build up of pressure in the abdomen in the later months as the growing baby causes the uterus to enlarge and push against the stomach. This, combined with hormonal factors, such as the effect of progesterone relaxing the upper sphincter muscle of the stomach, makes regurgitation much more likely.

Taking a herbal antacid remedy helps to bring relief. A number of these medicines are described on later pages. Drinking sips of milk also helps.

Oesophagitis may be described by the sufferer as a localised pressure or squeezing pain across the middle of the chest, which can radiate to the back.

Longstanding cases may develop a stricture, or partial blockage in the oesophagus which causes pain behind the breast bone after drinking hot liquids or acid foods. Constant difficulty in swallowing solid foods also suggests the development of a stricture.

Chapter 4

A Pain in the Chest

It is sometimes difficult for a person with hiatus hernia to know whether the chest pain they are suffering is due to the hernia or to some other cause — a heart condition, for example.

The pain arising from gastro-oesophageal reflux, more commonly in association with a sliding hiatus hernia, can cause a pain in the centre of the chest which is very much like angina.

Spasm of the oesophagus, related to reflux, may also cause central chest pain. There are a number of other painful conditions affecting the oesophagus which can also be mistaken for hiatus hernia.

With angina, the pain, like cramp, is due to a shortage of oxygen reaching the heart tissue. It is usually described as heavy or crushing, and it may radiate to the neck and jaw, or to the arms. It is more likely to be triggered by movement, particularly exercise or exertion. In someone who is resting, anginal pain tends never to last longer than a few minutes, whereas hiatal pain can last much longer.

People with osteoporosis or arthritic changes in the lower cervical or upper thoracic spine may also experience a referred pain which is felt in the chest. One way of identifying this pain, and distinguishing it from those caused by heart problems or a hernia, is that it can often be reproduced by making specific bodily movements. X-rays of the spine may or may not be helpful in diagnosis since most people over the age of fifty have degenerative changes in the spine but do not necessarily suffer from any specific symptoms as a result of them.

Chapter 5

About Achalasia

Achalasia is a condition which involves muscular spasm, but it refers not so much to an actual contraction of the tissues as the inability of the muscles to relax properly.

As a medical condition affecting the oesophagus it is sometimes known as cardiospasm, or achalasia of the cardia, and refers to a spasm of the muscular tissue of the sphincter where the oesophagus, or food pipe, passes through the diaphragm and enters the stomach.

The spasm causes an obstruction to food passing into the stomach. There is sometimes also an inflammation of the mucous membrane lining the oesophagus.

This condition, which can be mistaken for hiatus hernia in some patients, can occur at any age, but is more common in men between the ages of 30 and 50. On eating a meal, the food is felt to stick in the lower part of the oesophagus and pain may be felt behind the sternum.

Depending on the severity of the condition, the food may be cleared by vomiting, or it may gradually make its way into the stomach.

There is usually a rapid loss of weight to start with, but this may then stabilise.

The same symptoms could also be caused by a stricture or tumour in the oesophagus, so it is essential to confirm the diagnosis before any treatment is started. Indeed, any symptom affecting the oesophagus needs to be carefully investigated.

With achalasia a barium x-ray undertaken in hospital will show the barium collecting above the sphincter muscle, causing the oesophagus to dilate and twist like a coil. As more of the barium meal is taken, the obstruction may be overcome and some of the barium will pass into the stomach.

It is not clear exactly why the muscular tissue in the oesophagus fails to relax, but as it sometimes comes on quite suddenly there is a feeling that in some cases at least it may be associated with emotional shock.

Achalasia can exist for many years and keep the sufferer in a lowered state of health, or give rise to complications affecting the lungs. In order to reduce these risks, sufferers may often need to change their dietary habits.

Because of the difficulty that swallowed food has in passing into the stomach it is clear that an optimum diet must be followed in order to avoid weight loss. It is best to take small meals more often, selecting only one or two items at each sitting. High protein and energy foods, and fresh melt-in-the mouth foods, which are easily digested are usually favoured.

Surgical dilation of the muscular tissue has been resorted to in severe cases.

Chapter 6

Related Conditions

ANAEMIA

Anaemia may occur when hiatus hernia is accompanied by reflux oesophagitis. It is usually due to a slight but persistent haemorrhage from the damaged internal surfaces.

The blood travels down through the intestinal tract and is finally excreted in the stools. The presence of blood in the stools may not be obvious from a simple visual examination. However, it can be detected with a simple laboratory test.

The symptoms of anaemia due to chronic, insidious blood loss, include fatigue and general debility. There may also be breathlessness and cramping pains.

The anaemia is treated by healing the damaged internal tissues through modification of the diet towards soft fibre foods as described in Chapter 9, and by taking soothing herbal medicines. The health of the blood is rebuilt with these herbal medicines, plus iron and other minerals, preferably derived from natural sources.

I must emphasise that it is not sufficient just to take iron pills in a bid to treat anaemia without rectifying the cause of blood loss.

A blood test for anaemia forms part of the routine examination carried out in my practice and by similarly qualified herbal and naturopathic practitioners.

In young children, hiatus hernia would need to be suspected by the practitioner as a possible cause of anaemia as there may be no other indications that the condition is present.

SWALLOWING PROBLEMS

Nine out of ten people with reflux oesophagitis related to hiatus hernia have difficulty in swallowing food. This is known medically as dysphagia. Not being able to swallow is a distressing symptom and one which may also be associated with other more serious conditions, including cancer of the throat. It is essential, therefore, that any complaint of dysphagia be properly investigated.

Dysphagia is not always painful, but usually is when inflammation of the oesophagus is present. The pain is felt in the region of the breast bone.

VOMITING

The sight of blood is always worrying, particularly if it is vomited or coughed up, when a medical examination is essential. About one in six people with hiatus hernia mention that they have experienced such an attack or attacks. But about one in three lose traces of blood without being aware of it.

Hiatus hernia is a common cause of vomiting blood in pregnancy, but any such attack should always be thoroughly investigated to establish a definite diagnosis.

BREATHLESSNESS

Breathlessness occurs in hiatus hernia most commonly as a result of swallowing air, and is relieved by belching. But it may also occur because of occult blood loss (see Anaemia), or because the stomach becomes distended and presses on the lungs. In severe cases a lung may collapse causing extreme breathlessness, and demanding immediate medical attention.

Chapter 7

Starting Treatment

Herbalists and naturopaths would not advise strong drugs or surgery for hiatus hernia, except in severe cases. The surgery involved is not minor and carries a higher risk of an adverse outcome in older age groups.

If action is taken early there is much that the sufferer can do to alleviate the condition, and greatly reduce the risk of either surgery or drug treatment ever becoming necessary.

The most important step is a complete overhaul of one's diet. In most cases it is a faulty diet which is behind the development of the disease, so whatever other steps are taken, progress will never be as fast as when the diet is improved.

For details of the foods recommended turn to Chapter 9 on The Role of Diet.

OTHER MEASURES

Symptoms are generally worse when lying down in bed. So, to prevent acid seeping up from the stomach into the oesophagus through the incompetent sphincter at night, it is recommended that the head end of the bed be raised by four to six inches (or a little more if still considered comfortable) by placing blocks of wood under the legs.

This measure will be more effective if the last meal before bed has been completely digested. The next recommendation, therefore, is not to eat at bedtime. It is better if the last meal of the day is taken at least four hours before retiring.

It is also important not to overeat. Go for three or four small, but wholesome, meals a day and avoid eating between meals. Not only will this help to keep your weight down, but you might live longer. It has been found that people who eat sparingly tend to live longer — whether or not they have hiatus hernia.

Do not drink with food, particularly very hot or very cold drinks. Experience shows that dryish meals are best. Drink in between meals, preferably a herb tea that is also good for the digestion.

If you are overweight it is essential to lose the excess. I am not recommending any crash dieting regimes, but a sensible eating programme as outlined in this book, and a programme of gentle exercises, gentle because vigorous sports like squash have been blamed by many patients for causing the onset of their symptoms.

For relief of symptoms, such as heartburn and flatulence, herbal medicines that are naturally antacid, anti-inflammatory, anti-flatulent and soothing, should be used in preference to drugs.

If you are taking drugs for hiatus hernia or another unrelated condition, you should be aware of any side effects that they may induce. A selection of medicines commonly prescribed for hiatus hernia as well as some that may act adversely on the sphincter muscle at the top of the stomach, are listed in Chapter 8. It is part of naturopathic medicine to wean patients off inappropriate drug therapy. Indeed, there are few naturopaths who have not achieved "miracle cures" simply by taking their patients off of unnecessary medication. The reader is advised, however, not to stop any medicines without proper advice.

Smoking is not allowed (not even one a day). The nicotine in cigarettes is a drug that not only increases acid production, but interferes with the function of the sphincter muscles. Herbal medicines are available from herbal practitioners to help you give up smoking if this is a problem.

Coughs must be treated actively with herbal medication. Continual coughing causes physical trauma which can initially cause, or aggravate hiatus hernia.

Tight clothing is claimed by some specialists to be a cause of hiatus hernia, but my opinion is that this is unlikely, although it could aggravate the condition. Therefore, clothes like corsets are best avoided and braces are better than belts.

BABIES

Treating babies with hiatus hernia is very difficult as they suffer symptoms when they are lying down. Parents of such infants need specialist advice from paediatricians. The babies may need to sleep in specially-adapted cots which keep them more upright and be fed on thickened liquid foods.

Fortunately, in most cases the condition improves when the child begins to walk, but surgery may be necessary in cases where there is no improvement or where complications develop.

Chapter 8

Treatment with Drugs

In milder cases of hiatus hernia, the individual may have been prescribed any of a number of simple drugs to ease the symptoms, or, indeed, be using over-the-counter medicines.

Doctors have a wide range of remedies from which to choose in treating hiatus hernia, particularly for dealing with complaints like heartburn, acidity and reflux.

In more serious cases, for example, where the oesophagus has become ulcerated, it is usually necessary to resort to more powerful medicines, many of which have been available only in recent years.

Among the medicines most commonly prescribed by doctors are antacids and reflux suppressants.

This chapter gives information on some of these drugs and, where relevant, any undesirable effects which may be associated with them.

There are also a few drugs prescribed for other diseases which may aggravate some of the symptoms of hiatus hernia.

It is not intended to alarm anyone who may be taking any of these medicines; rather it is hoped that the individual will be more informed about their effects.

It is emphasised that individuals react differently to drugs and will not necessarily suffer any side-effects. Do not stop any drug treatment prescribed by a doctor without proper medical advice.

SODIUM BICARBONATE:

Sodium bicarbonate, or baking soda, is used in numerous over-the-counter and prescription medicines and is taken by millions of people for its antacid properties. It quickly relieves indigestion due to increased acidity in the stomach, and helps to allay pain in hiatus hernia and oesophageal inflammation. However, once in the stomach it produces carbon dioxide gas which causes "burping" and may mislead the person who is taking it into thinking that it was the wind that was causing the pain.

Naturopaths are unhappy about the regular use of "bicarb" as it can alter the acid-alkaline balance of the blood, towards alkaline and cause a condition known as alkalosis. It can also be a cause of kidney stones.

Because it contains sodium, "bicarb" is contraindicated in those who have high blood pressure as sodium tends to hold fluid in the system. For the same reason it is not suitable for people who suffer from fluid retention or oedema as it may exacerbate the condition. Others who should avoid sodium bicarbonate are people with heart or kidney disease and the elderly.

ALUMINIUM HYDROXIDE:

This is a slowish-acting remedy for acidity. It is incorporated into prescription medicines for heartburn, hiatus hernia, acid reflux and inflammation of the oesophagus.

There has been much speculation in recent years about a possible association between aluminium and pre-senile dementia, or Alzheimer's disease. It has been argued that indigestion remedies are currently the chief source of "dietary" aluminium, and that they may be contributing to this degenerative brain disease. Another source would be the use of aluminium cookware.

Despite a reasonable amount of epidemiological evidence, there is as yet no absolute proof that aluminium is associated with Alzheimer's disease. However, naturopaths would be extremely cautious about the use of this ingredient in indigestion remedies.

One of the main side-effects associated with aluminium hydroxide is constipation. It can also interfere with both the absorption of vitamins and phosphate, an important constituent of bone.

MAGNESIUM HYDROXIDE

A slow-acting antacid, sometimes known as cream of magnesia, this magnesium salt can cause diarrhoea. A combination of aluminium hydroxide and magnesium hydroxide, together with other ingredients, are often prescribed for hiatus hernia. It may be thought that the constipating effects of the former cancels out the bowel looseness created by the latter. In practice this may not be the case.

Magnesium is contraindicated in people with serious kidney disease.

MAGNESIUM TRISILICATE

Although relatively slow-acting as an antacid, it gives relief over a longer period. It mops up pepsin, a fermenting agent found in the gastric juice.

CALCIUM CARBONATE:

A common ingredient in medicines for gastric hyperacidity. Unlike sodium bicarbonate it does not interfere with the blood's acid-alkaline ratio, but it tends to cause constipation.

This is another remedy not advised for regular use as it may lead to hypercalcaemia — a too high level of calcium in the blood which can depress muscular and nervous functions.

Although calcium deficiency is far more common than calcium excess, the body's requirements for this mineral are best obtained from a wholesome diet, including skimmed milk, rather than from an indigestion tablet.

Calcium excess is more likely in people who are drinking a lot of milk, taking a calcium supplement and indigestion tablets containing calcium carbonate. They may suffer muscular weakness and headaches as well as gastro-intestinal symptoms such as constipation, abdominal pain and feeling nauseous.

ALGINIC ACID

Pharmaceutical companies utilise seaweed in their medicines. Green algae from the sea are used pharmaceutically in the manufacture of alginic acid, and from that, compounds such as magnesium or sodium alginate. They help to break down and disperse the ingredients of tablets once they are in the stomach.

When sodium bicarbonate is incorporated in a tablet, carbon dioxide is released and keeps the alginic acid floating above it. This forms a barrier to stomach acid and thus prevents symptoms like heartburn.

CIMETIDINE

This is classified as an acid inhibitor. It works by blocking the secretion of acid by gastric cells. The philosophy is that where there is no acid there is no pain, particularly in conditions like peptic ulcer. It is also indicated for symptoms arising from acid reflux.

Unfortunately, it can give rise to a number of unpleasant side-effects, including dizziness, mental confusion, skin rash, loose bowel and weariness. It can cause liver upset and, in men, excessive growth of the breast area.

CISAPRIDE MONOHYDRATE

A drug that improves the muscular movements of stomach and oesophagus and so indicated in reflux and hiatus hernia where decreased sphincter tone is a problem. It is not recommended in pregnancy or the elderly, or where there is kidney or liver disease. It may cause diarrhoea, stomach rumblings and cramp in the abdominal muscles. On rare occasions cisapride monohydrate has been associated with convulsions.

NIZATIDINE

An acid inhibitor like cimetidine, prescribed for the symptoms of acid reflux. It should not be taken during pregnancy or while breast feeding. It may cause a skin rash, sweats, sleepiness and liver disturbances.

METOCLOPRAMIDE

Indicated in hiatus hernia, acid reflux and inflammation of the oesophagus, metoclopramide helps prevent reflux by acting on the sphincter muscles of the stomach. Drowsiness and diarrhoea may occur, but modern sustained-release formulations have tended to reduce these effects. It should not be taken during pregnancy, or while breast feeding.

GAVISCON

One of the most commonly prescribed medicines for heartburn, hiatus hernia and symptoms due to acid reflux. It combines sodium bicarbonate, alginic acid, magnesium trisilicate, and dried aluminium hydroxide gel.

OMEPRAZOLE

A new class of drug used in severe inflammatory disease of the oesophagus. It may cause headaches, bowel upsets, skin rashes and nausea.

CARBENOXOLONE SODIUM

This semi-synthetic derivative of liquorice is used for healing ulcers, but it is also indicated for oesophageal reflux and inflammation. Unfortunately, it may cause water retention, high blood pressure, and lowered blood potassium levels. As potassium is vital to the heart it is contraindicated in those with heart conditions: indeed, it may interact adversely with the heart drug digoxin. It is not advised for the elderly, or to be taken in pregnancy.

BETHANECHOL CHLORIDE

This drug acts on the sphincter muscles, rather like metoclopramide, to prevent acid reflux, but it can produce side-effects, including cramping pains in the abdomen, vomiting, visual disturbance, bladder frequency and sweating. People with asthma, epilepsy, thyroid conditions, and low blood pressure are among those not advised to use it.

OTHER DRUGS

Theophylline, used in the treatment of asthma, relaxes the muscular tissue of the lung, but may also over-relax the sphincter muscle guarding the oesophagus and aggravate any acid reflux.

Similar caution applies to some of the modern calcium channel blocker drugs used in the treatment of high blood pressure, hormone treatment with progesterone, and the tranquilliser, diazepam.

Chapter 9

The Role of Diet

The role of diet in the cause and treatment of hiatus hernia is still, surprisingly, a controversial topic.

The general consensus of those who have investigated the causes and treated the disease over many years is that the cause is related to a high-calorie, fibre-deficient diet.

Therefore, the initial treatment must be to prevent any further deterioration in the physical condition of the patient by instituting a diet rich in fibrous foods.

However, just to state that lack of fibre in the diet causes the disease is a gross over-simplification, because the physical effects of fibre-depleted food are numerous.

For example, lack of fibre in the diet may cause constipation, and one theory has been that *straining* to produce a stool when constipated increases pressure in the abdomen to such a degree that the stomach is pushed through the diaphragm (see Chapter 10).

Another suggestion is that the sliding hiatus hernia is due to *over-eating*. Too much food in the stomach, whether fibrous or not, particularly when one is not really hungry, slows down digestion. Many people feel that when they are hungry they "could eat a horse", but when full, eating just a mouthful more creates gastric discomfort, including acid reflux. A hernia, it is suggested, does not cause the acid, but is a result of excessive acid production.

My belief is that over-consumption of refined carbo-hydrate foods, which are fibre-depleted, has an overall degenerating effect on the body, including stomach function. This becomes the *predisposing* cause of hiatus hernia.

The syndrome then may be quite easily triggered off by even a small exertion, but particularly in those who are elderly, have constipation, or who are overweight.

This is much the same as saying that cold winter weather does not cause bronchitis. Although bronchitis is common in winter, the lungs of the potential bronchitic are already in a poor condition. Winter is merely the trigger, or exciting cause, of the disease.

DIETARY TREATMENT

Many practitioners who associate lack of dietary fibre with hiatus hernia fail to appreciate that there is more than one fibre in food and that all fibres do not suit all people.

Therefore, merely recommending a high-fibre diet is just not good enough.

I do not, for example, recommend people with hiatus hernia, to transform their diet by eating nuts, beans and sprouts, although this is recommended in some health books. On the contrary I would advise that these foods be avoided.

Neither do I recommend fasting for this condition. Fasting is an important naturopathic method of treatment in many diseases and would not be contraindicated when necessary, for example, where an infection is present. But I believe that the digestive system functions better and heals faster if it receives the appropriate foods, because they have a natural, soothing and massaging effect on the surfaces of the stomach as they pass through.

Over the past 20 years my advice has been to greatly increase the amount of soft fibre in the diet. Foods that can be mashed, such as boiled potato and carrots are ideal. They are rich in fibre, but not irritating to the stomach.

Easily digested foods, such as fish and cottage cheese, provide adequate protein, and are to be preferred to red meat, which takes a while to digest.

Pulpy foods, such as melons and avocados, soothe the stomach and are far better than stringy foods.

Foods which are usually eaten whole, but which may have tough skins, like tomatoes, are best peeled first. Foods containing pips are also best eaten only in small quantities, at least in the early stages of treatment.

In general, the diet should not contain any processed foods or refined carbohydrates — white bread, white sugar, white rice and white pasta, or confectionery. Stick to natural whole foods whenever possible. There is no evidence that fresh whole food will make a hiatus hernia worse. Indeed, the whole body will respond better and one's general health will improve.

Eat easily-digested salad foods, like beetroot, tender organically-grown vegetables and fruits, and drink diluted fruit and vegetable juices and herb teas. Alcohol, tea and coffee are banned.

Among the foods to avoid are those that cause flatulence, such as onions, beans, peas, cauliflower and raw cabbage, and hard, splintery foods like crispbread. Fried food, rich fatty foods and condiments — salt, vinegar and pickles — are also best left alone.

In summary, eat small meals, more often, but eat only when hungry; confine yourself to low calorie, soft high-fibre foods. Thus, wholewheat bread and wholewheat cereals, which are soft fibres, are preferable to cereals with hard fibres, such as oats.

Very hot and very cold drinks and food, long drinks and drinking with meals will upset the stomach at this time.

For those who possess a juicer, a cocktail made from equal parts of apples, carrots and beetroot, is recommended. Drink about a wineglassful two or three times a day.

Chapter 10

*Ease the Strain —
Eliminate Constipation*

It is essential for the successful treatment of hiatus hernia to eradicate any tendency to constipation.

Where constipation exists there is always the risk of straining to produce a stool, and this not only exacerbates the underlying condition, but may have been the major factor in the appearance of the disease in the first place.

Naturopaths and herbalists have written extensively for years on the role that diet plays in chronic constipation; and the importance of dietary fibre has been consistently emphasised.

People with hiatus hernia should follow carefully the advice on diet given in this book. They cannot expect their constipation to be resolved by half-hearted attempts. Simply switching from a sugary, refined cereal to a bowl of bran flakes is not enough.

Straining increases the abdominal pressure much more than that in the chest and some researchers believe that this is enough to cause the stomach sphincter to herniate.

A more normal bowel motion and a daily habit will be achieved only if an increase in a soft fibre, such as wholewheat cereals, is accompanied by an increase in fluid intake.

Failure to take note of this may simply result in the stools becoming harder and more difficult to pass.

Patients whose bowels do not improve after changing from white to wholemeal bread, and so on, should increase other sources of fibre in the diet such as fruit and vegetables and brown rice and pasta.

They should also realise that many drugs have a constipating effect.

Opiates, iron tablets, certain antidepressants and antacids can all reduce the natural movements of the intestinal tract.

In the early stages of treatment it may be necessary to take a herbal aperient to aid the bowel movement.

A remedy, such as Californian buckthorn (*Cascara sagrada*) will be found to be very effective. The tincture, or fluid extract, has a bitter taste, but specially-coated tablets which are easier to take are available from medical herbalists.

This remedy does not purge the bowel or cause cramping pains and increasing doses will not be found to be necessary.

The remedy can be taken at bedtime for about ten days and then the dose gradually tapered off and finally stopped altogether. One should not become reliant on it.

Chapter 11

Favourite Herbal Remedies

There are a number of individual remedies that tend to be used more frequently than others in the treatment of hiatus hernia, because they have been found over time to give the best results in the majority of cases. These remedies can be regarded as "specifics" and are described below.

However, as symptoms may vary from person to person, the general digestive system remedies described in later chapters should also be considered.

THE GOLDEN REMEDY

The remedy I am about to describe is worth its weight in gold. It is the medicine derived from the rhizome of *Hydrastis canadensis*, known commonly as goldenseal. It is not an inexpensive item: it is used extensively all over the world by herbalists and naturopaths and demand for it has ensured the suppliers of a high price on the herb markets. In its wild form it is has virtually disappeared and so we now have to use the plant cultivated by farmers.

Why is this herb so sought after? It has been described as the king of all herbs used in the treatment of the mucous membranes — the tissues that line the body organs. And it is a leading agent in the treatment of gastric disease. In herbal practice we could not be without it. Sore inflamed tissues respond remarkably well to it — even the surface of the eye, which is treated with a lotion made from the powdered root. Goldenseal also used to be incorporated into ointments to soothe red and inflamed eyelids and was highly effective.

Goldenseal is used in the treatment of hiatus hernia not only because it is a healer of ulcerated and inflamed tissue, but also because it is an excellent gastric tonic, an anti-dyspeptic and anti-ulcer remedy.

Who do we thank for this? First of all the medicine men of the Red Indian people and then the early American herbal doctors who added to the knowledge gained from them. Until the late 1940s it was listed officially in the British Pharmacopoeia.

The Red Indians used it to paint their skin gold and found it healed up any skin troubles, such as ulcers and sores. The lesson learned was that the epithelium of the skin is the same as the epithelium lining the mouth, throat and intestinal canal — thus goldenseal works as well inside as out. Its only drawback is that it has a bitter taste.

However, it is so effective that it is taken only in small doses, or better still, small amounts are combined with other remedies. It is contra-indicated in pregnancy.

Tinctures and fluid extracts are made by herbalists, but the powdered root can be used to make an infusion — take in teaspoonful doses or less, or put a teaspoonful of infusion into a herb tea and add honey to taste.

THE SOOTHER

Herbalists have praised the healing virtues of the inner bark of *Ulmus fulva*, the slippery elm tree, ever since the discovery of America. It is among the most useful of all herbal medicines and was used extensively by the Red Indians in the north and by the native tribes in South America.

The bark is powdered and made into a drink or into tablets which have a soothing effect on all tissues with which they come into contact.

Ulmus is the old Latin name for the elm tree, of which there are a number of varieties. The bark of the common English elm, which has unfortunately suffered attacks by Dutch elm disease, is also soothing if used as a poultice, but is not considered to be as effective as slippery elm.

To make a mucilaginous drink from the powder of *Ulmus fulva,* you should use one teaspoonful to a pint of boiling water, or milk, which is slowly poured on to it, and stirred constantly as if making a sauce. If the mixture becomes too lumpy strain it before use. The taste can be improved by adding a pinch of powdered nutmeg or cinnamon. Two or three cups a day, or more if required, may be taken.

Simmering the bark in water for an hour as if making a decoction will produce a more mucilaginous liquid, or gruel.

The bark is not only healing and soothing, but also nutritious when it is known as slippery elm food. It can be given to invalids and will be nourishing when other foods cannot be taken.

It will be found to be particularly valuable in severe cases of hiatus hernia where the oesophagus has become ulcerated.

Tablets are available from herbalists. Two or three are chewed and swallowed at meal times.

THE ANTACID

The heartburn associated with hiatus hernia can be eased, depending on severity, with what has become known among herbalists as the herbal bicarbonate of soda.

A gentle, healing herb, meadowsweet (*Spiraea ulmaria*) is a good first-line treatment for acidity, eructations, heartburn, and other digestive diseases.

It is also known by one or two other common names, including Queen of the Meadow and Lady of the Meadow.

It is probably most effective when used as an infusion.

One can use the white flowers, which resemble the garden varieties of Spiraea, the chopped leaves, or the whole chopped herb, excluding the root.

The flowers, which appear in early summer are pleasantly aromatic and are often preferred.

To make the infusion steep one ounce of the flowers in 20 fluid ounces (one pint) of boiling water in a covered jug for about 10 minutes. Then strain the liquid and take it in doses of two fluid ounces (about a wineglassful) as necessary. Tinctures are prescribed by herbalists.

Meadowsweet helps to normalise the production of the stomach acids if used over a period of time. In this case it is used at times when there are no symptoms present. Take one or two small wineglassfuls of the infusion every day.

It may be combined, when not contraindicated, with liquorice, which is anti-inflammatory, and dandelion root, which improves overall digestion by stimulating liver and gall bladder function.

Simmer half an ounce each of liquorice and dandelion root in 30 fluid ounces of water for about 20 minutes and then remove from the heat. Add half an ounce of meadowsweet and a quarter-ounce of peppermint herb. Infuse until the liquid cools and add honey to taste. Take in doses of from two teaspoonfuls to two fluid ounces three or four times a day, according to age and severity of the condition.

THE EMOLLIENT

An emollient is a remedy that softens and soothes. One of the best is Marshmallow, which is an essential herb in the treatment of hiatus hernia, particularly where there is much inflammation and irritation. Its official name, *Althaea officinalis,* means to cure, while mallow means to soften.

It thrives in damp meadows and on banks of rivers and was always grown in gardens in former times because of its medicinal properties.

As all of the medicinal properties are soluble in water it is an ideal remedy for domestic use either as an infusion of the leaves or a decoction of the root — both of which are available from herbalists.

To make an infusion use one ounce of the leaves, which are picked from the plant just as the flowers are coming into bloom. Add them to one pint of boiling water and allow to cool. Strain and add honey or orange juice. The dose is two fluid ounces three of four times a day, or combine it with slippery elm.

Take half an ounce of each and simmer in 40 fluid ounces of water until the total is reduced to 30 fluid ounces. Strain the liquid and add honey to taste. The mixture may be taken in doses of two fluid ounces three or four times a day.

THE HEALER

An ancient medicinal herb, and one of the more pleasant, is *Glycyrrhiza glabra,* or liquorice. Few remedies can equal its ability to heal damaged gastrointestinal mucosa. This is why extractions and modifications of it are used to produce modern anti-ulcer drugs.

Added to herbal mixtures it improves their medicinal virtues and taste.

As a demulcent it is particularly soothing to the gastrointestinal tract.

The infusion of one ounce of bruised root, with bark removed, in one pint of boiling water heals ulcerated tissue. Most people with hiatus hernia will find it helpful. Drink a wineglassful two or three times a day. A strong decoction of the root will relieve constipation.

Unfortunately liquorice is not good for everybody as it may exacerbate fluid retention. It is, therefore, contraindicated in people who suffer from high blood pressure.

Chapter 12

Herbal Preparations

Herbal medicines are now widely available from health stores and from other retail outlets, as well as on private prescription from medical herbalists. But "teas" made at home, from herbs supplied by herbalists, may be equally effective.

Most medical herbalists would agree that, where the medicinal properties of a herb are soluble in water, infusions and decoctions are probably the best way to take them.

Do not take herbal medicines at the same time as taking medicines from the doctor without appropriate advice as there is the possibility of an interaction.

INFUSIONS

Infusions, also known as teas or tisanes, are usually made with the softer parts of the plant, such as the flowers or leaves. These are chopped finely and about an ounce placed in a jug, preferably one with a close fitting lid. Pour a pint (20 fluid ounces) of boiling water on to the herb and cover the jug. Infuse the herb for 10 to 15 minutes, stirring occasionally. When ready strain off the tea. The usual dose range is from half to two fluid ounces — that is no more than a small wineglassful — three times a day. If the medicine is to be taken on a long-term basis a maximum of half an ounce to one pint of water is usually recommended.

DECOCTIONS

Decoctions are more suitable for the harder parts of the plant, such as the bark, roots and berries. To every ounce of the plant material, which is best ground down into a rough powder, or finely chopped, pour on 1½ pints (30 fluid ounces) of cold water, cover and allow to stand overnight. Then bring to the boil and simmer for 20 minutes, or until there is a pint (20 fluid ounces) of water left. Strain and drink half to two fluid ounces two or three times a day.

Infusions and decoctions can also be made in a coffee percolator.

TINCTURES

These are used when the medicinal properties are either destroyed by heat, or not sufficiently soluble in water. The herb is steeped (macerated) in a mixture (known as the menstruum) of alcohol and cold water — usually a minimum of 20 per cent pure alcohol — for at least two weeks before being pressed out and filtered ready for use. The tinctures prescribed by medical herbalists are made commercially with pure alcohol for which a government licence is necessary. They may also undergo the process of maceration and filtration several times in order to strengthen the tincture and to reduce the final alcohol content to a minimum.

For home use tinctures can be made with brandy, but this is a rather an expensive process. However, the preparation is much stronger than a simple infusion or decoction, the ratio being 1:5 — one ounce of the herb to five fluid ounces of menstruum. Most tinctures need a 25 per cent proportion of alcohol to water. Dosage ranges from 10-40 drops (½ml-2ml), except for the more potent remedies. The advantage of tinctures is that they are more convenient to use and they keep well.

Some herbalists, including myself, prefer tinctures made in the ratio of 1:3 — one ounce of herb to three ounces of menstruum. On filtration the amount of tincture recovered is made equal to the original amount, that is three ounces, by making up the amount with further menstruum, or by remaceration.

FLUID EXTRACTS

Strong tinctures, or fluid extracts, are made by reducing the final amount recovered. This is achieved by evaporation on a very low heat for several hours using a water bath, or double saucepan. An official fluid extract is one that contains the equivalent of one ounce of herb to every fluid ounce of extract (a ratio of 1:1) and contains an adequate amount of alcohol to preserve it.

LOTIONS

Medicinal preparations such as lotions, mouth washes, gargles and douches can be made from infusions. They are best filtered after straining off the herb.

ESSENTIAL OILS

Pure oils extracted from plants are extremely potent — and toxic in overdose — and should not be taken internally without adequate knowledge of the individual remedy. They are mainly used externally and in dilution by rubbing on to the skin.

Many of them tend to be antifungal and antibiotic in action. One drop of peppermint oil dropped on to the tongue is so strong it makes the eyes water. The potency of essential oils can be seen from the effect of just adding a few drops into bath water. Prescribed correctly, plant oils are a useful addition to the herbal dispensary. Appropriate remedies can be diluted one part in a hundred parts of water and used in douches.

INFUSED OILS

These are quite different from essential oils. Herbs, such as Calendula and Comfrey are steeped in a bland oil, such as olive oil, in a warm place — traditionally in the sun — for at least two weeks so that the medicinal properties are infused into the oil. They are then strained ready for use and, therefore, the strength may vary. One can keep repeating the infusion process by adding more herb to the oil and setting aside for a further time. A practitioner would use an infused oil of comfrey, for example, for deep massage to the abdomen to improve circulation and to help remove toxic waste from the colon.

Chapter 13

Some Recommended Herbs

Herbal medicines have a long history of use in the treatment of stomach and intestinal diseases.

This section contains a description of botanic remedies frequently prescribed by herbalists to alleviate the symptoms associated with hiatus hernia and other digestive disorders. It also includes remedies which have a general toning effect on the whole body. Herbalists and naturopaths always treat their patients as whole people rather than as a collection of components.

Do remember that caution with all medicines, including herbs, is advised during pregnancy. While most are safe, a few are contraindicated and, therefore, should be taken only under the supervision of a qualified practitioner. The same caution applies to the treatment of babies and young children.

Some herbs may be available only on a private prescription from a medical herbalist.

Agar-Agar
GELIDIUM AMANSII

Also known as Japanese isinglass

Where found Japan

Appearance Seaweed

Part used Dried strips of the plant

Therapeutic use A vegetarian jelly is made from the mucilaginous strips which is both soothing and nutritious. Ideal for those with stomach conditions where food intake is restricted.

Prepared as Jelly which may be flavoured with lemon, or other fruits.

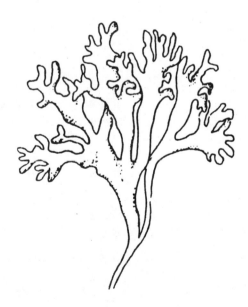

Agar-Agar

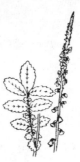

Agrimony
AGRIMONIA EUPATORIA

Also known as	Church steeples
Where found	Throughout northern Europe
Appearance	A strong growing herb with green/grey leaves covered with soft hairs. Flowers are small and yellow on long slender spikes.
Part used	Herb
Therapeutic uses	A good general tonic for the whole system. The dried leaves when infused are useful in treating simple diarrhoea and general intestinal debility, and to help prevent tissue wasting due to malabsorption. One of several herbs used to treat anaemic conditions. Agrimony also improves skin function, helping to clear skin eruptions, pimples and blotches.
Prepared as	Infusion, tincture.

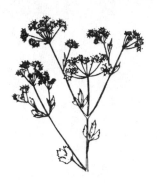

Aniseed
PIMPINELLA ANISUM

Also known as	Anise.
Where found	Grown in southern Europe, North Africa, India and South America.
Appearance	White flowering garden herb with feathery leaves, growing to about 50cm high.
Part used	Seeds.
Therapeutic uses	A valuable remedy for flatulence and colic.
Prepared as	Powder, infusion, tincture.

Arrowroot
MARANTA ARUNDINACEA

Where found	West Indies
Appearance	Tall herbaceous plant

Arrowroot

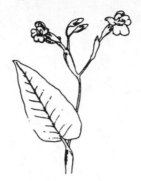

Part used Rhizome

Therapeutic uses Arrowroot is nutritious, healing and soothing to stomach and bowels and will not upset when the stomach is irritated. Boil two or three teaspoonfuls of the powder in a pint of water to make a gruel. Sweeten to taste with honey and flavour with a pinch of cinnamon powder or fruit juice. It may also be combined with Slippery Elm.

Prepared as Powder

Bayberry
MYRICA CERIFERA

Also known as	Candle Berry
Where found	United States
Appearance	Shrub up to 8ft high with shiny leaves and globular berries
Parts used	Bark

Therapeutic uses	A valuable tonic and cleanser for the whole system. It improves circulation and removes catarrh from the stomach. Indicated where there is anaemia. Women will find that this remedy improves the blood supply to the uterus and is useful for treating uterine prolapse.
Prepared as	Powder, fluid extract, tincture, decoction.

Black Cohosh
CIMICIFUGA RACEMOSA

Also known as	Squaw Root
Where found	United States and Canada
Appearance	A tall herbaceous plant with white feathery flowers.
Parts used	Rhizome
Therapeutic uses	A general blood purifier and nervine tonic, with antispasmodic and sedative properties. It is anti-flatuent, but mainly has a reputation as a woman's remedy, particularly in improving menstrual flow. Use in small doses as large doses may cause nausea and vomiting. This herb should not be taken during pregnancy.
Prepared as	Infusion, decoction, syrup, tincture.

Cardamom
ELETTARIA CARDAMOMUM

Also known as   Malabar Cardamom

Where found   Ceylon and India

Appearance   Forest plant with large smooth, dark green leaves and small yellowish flowers

Part used   Fruits, seeds and oil

Therapeutic uses   An aromatic herb mainly used in the treatment of flatulence and to improve the digestion.

Prepared as   Powder, liquid extract, tincture.

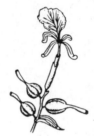

Cardamom

Chamomile, wild
MATRICARIA CHAMOMILLA

Also known as   German chamomile

Where found   Corn fields in Europe

Appearance   Herb with small cushion-like flowers in profusion

Part used   Flowers

Therapeutic uses   A valuable gastro-intestinal tonic and stimulating nervine, with carminative, antispasmodic and anti-inflammatory properties. It reduces flatulence and abdominal distension and eases colicky pains and spasms in the colon.

Continual daily use is indicated where there is inflammation. A chamomile poultice helps to allay pain.

Prepared as   Infusion, poultice, tincture.

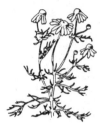

Wild Chamomile

Chamomile, common
ANTHEMIS NOBILIS

Also known as	Belgian chamomile
Where found	A favourite garden herb, abundant in France and Belgium, but widely cultivated.
Appearance	A herb resembling a large daisy with white flowers and yellow centres.
Parts used	Flowers and herb
Therapeutic uses	An antispasmodic indicated in stomach and intestinal disorders.

Very useful in heartburn, simple indigestion, flatulence, colic, and debilitated states of the colon. Also for simple diarrhoea in children. It is widely prescribed for nervous and hysterical conditions.

Prepared as   Infusion (chamomile tea), fluid extract, tincture.

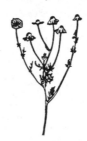

Common Chamomile

Cinnamon
CINNAMOMUM ZEYLANICUM

Where found	A native plant of Ceylon
Appearance	A tree growing up to 30ft high in sandy soils.
Part used	Bark
Therapeutic uses	A pleasantly aromatic herb with carminative, antiseptic, and astringent properties. An effective remedy for vomiting and nausea, and will give relief in flatulence and diarrhoea.
Prepared as	Oil, medicinal water, tincture, powder.

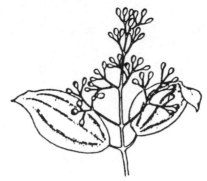

Clary
SALVIA SCLAREA

Also known as	Christ's Eye and Clary Sage
Where found	Common garden plant
Appearance	Similar to common sage with blue or white flowers
Parts used	Herb, seeds and essential oil
Therapeutic uses	It can be used for digestive problems in combination with chamomile where an antispasmodic is called for. Useful in colic and painful menstruation. Its main use has been for ophthalmic conditions (clary eye = clear eye). The essential oil is intoxicating, which led to it being regarded as an aphrodisiac.
Prepared as	Infusion and mucilage. Contraindicated for internal use in pregnancy.

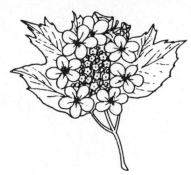

Cramp Bark
VIBURNUM OPULUS

Also known as	Snowball tree, Guelder rose
Where found	Europe and the United States
Appearance	Strong-growing bush with white ball-shaped flowers.
Part used	Bark.
Therapeutic uses	Cramp bark, as its name suggests, is an antispasmodic. It is also an excellent nervine. It gives relief in gastrointestinal colic.
Prepared as	Decoction and tincture.

Cranesbill
GERANIUM MACULATUM

Also known as	Wild geranium
Where found	United States

Appearance	Shrubby small herb with blue flowers. The seed pod resembles a crane's bill.
Parts used	Herb and root
Therapeutic uses	This remedy is indicated where there are ulcerated and mucous conditions of the stomach and intestines, particularly if the bowels are loose and there is a catarrhal discharge and bleeding. A useful treatment for piles.
Prepared as	Infusion of herb, decoction of root, powder, tincture

Echinacea
ECHINACEA ANGUSTIFOLIA

Also known as	Cone flower
Where found	American prairies
Appearance	Herb of medium height
Part used	Rhizome
Therapeutic uses	Natural antibiotic, antiseptic and alterative. Helps to clear the blood of toxic material. Improves appetite and digestion. Good when anaemia is present. Used in ulcerative conditions of the stomach and duodenum to keep the tissues clean. Can be combined with small amounts of goldenseal.
Prepared as	Decoction and tincture.

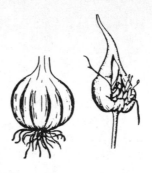

Garlic
ALLIUM SATIVUM

Where found	Universally cultivated
Appearance	Similar to a shallot
Part used	Bulb
Therapeutic uses	Not everyone with hiatus hernia will find that garlic agrees with them. However, it is useful for the treatment of dyspepsia and flatulence and it is a powerful antiseptic. It also reduces cholesterol in the blood. Try the juice or oil first.
Prepared as	Powder, oil (in capsules), juice, tablets and tincture.

Gentian
GENTIANA LUTEA

Also known as	Yellow Gentian
Where found	Alpine plant in Europe
Appearance	A hardy herbaceous perennial bearing clusters of large orange-yellow flowers.

Part used	Root
Therapeutic uses	One of the finest tonics for the stomach and intestines. It is very bitter to the taste even when greatly diluted, but it boosts appetite and aids digestion. Often prescribed when there is a general debility and jaundice. A useful remedy for dyspepsia. It is better to combine small doses of the medicine with an aromatic herb such as Cardamoms to help camouflage the bitter taste.
Prepared as	Tincture and powder (use up to a quarter of a teaspoonful infused in a cupful of boiling water and sweetened with honey).

Ginger
ZINGIBER OFFICINALE

Where found	West Indies and China
Appearance	About one metre high with glossy aromatic leaves.
Part used	Rhizome
Therapeutic uses	An excellent remedy for nausea and indigestion. Ginger is mainly used as a carminative — it reduces flatulence and distension and eases painful intestinal spasms. It also reduces fermentation in the bowel.
Prepared as	Powder, syrup, tablets and tincture.

Goldenseal
HYDRASTIS CANADENSIS

Also known as	Yellow root
Where found	Cultivated in North America
Appearance	Tall-growing herb with disagreeable odour
Part used	Rhizome
Therapeutic uses	A most important herb in herbal medicine. Excellent for treating diseases affecting the stomach. It is particularly soothing to the epithelium — the skin surface both outside and inside the body, including mouth, throat, stomach and intestinal lining. It is antiseptic, antifungal, laxative and purifies the blood. As a tonic it helps those with irritable and inflammatory conditions of the stomach and colon. It is indicated in most digestive disorders.
Prepared as	Decoction, powder, tincture. Use small doses only. Contraindicated in pregnancy.

Hops
HUMULUS LUPULUS

Where found	Cultivated in most parts of the world.
Appearance	A climbing vine

Hops

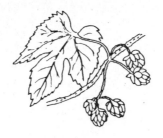

Part used	Strobiles
Therapeutic uses	A nervine tonic and sedative mainly used in combination with other remedies for indigestion and as a liver and gall bladder remedy. It allays pain and promotes restful sleep. Indicated in anaemic conditions.

Lady's Slipper
CYPRIPEDIUM PUBESCENS

Also known as	Nerve Root
Where found	Europe and the United States.
Appearance	A delicate wild orchid at present in short supply and, therefore, highly expensive. Attempts to grow it commercially for

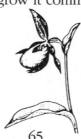

Lady's Slipper

medicinal use have not been very successful so far.

Parts used	Rhizome
Therapeutic uses	A most effective nervine used to allay disorders of a nervous origin, including emotional tension. It helps to induce natural sleep. It is also antispasmodic and relaxing.
Prepared as	Powder, decoction, fluid extract and tincture.

Lemon Balm
MELISSA OFFICINALIS

Also known as	Sweet Balm
Where found	A common garden herb
Appearance	It belongs to the nettle family to which it bears some resemblance, but has a strong lemon smell.
Parts used	Leaves, whole herb.
Therapeutic uses	Carminative. A useful and safe remedy for the stomach. It relieves flatulence and gastric upsets. Indicated when there is anaemia. It has antifungal properties and is also indicated in fevers. The hot infusion will induce sweating. An infusion of the leaves (one ounce to one pint of boiling water) can be drunk as required.

Lemon Balm

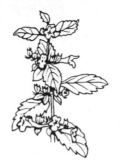

Marshmallow
ALTHAEA OFFICINALIS

Also known as	Schloss tea
Where found	Throughout Europe
Appearance	A strong-growing herb usually found in watery places
Parts used	Leaves and root
Therapeutic uses	An emollient and demulcent; soothing to the stomach and intestinal tract. Used in irritable and ulcerative conditions.
Prepared as	Infusion (of leaves), decoction (of root), syrup and tincture.

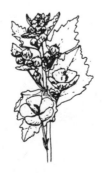

Marshmallow

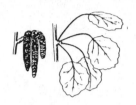

Poplar
POPULUS TREMULOIDES

Also known as	Quaking aspen
Where found	North America and Europe
Appearance	A large tree
Parts used	Bark
Therapeutic uses	A tonic that improves appetite and digestion and helps to dispel flatulence. A useful medicine to take during convalescence following a fever. It is indicated in diarrhoea. Poplar has also been found to be beneficial in cases of muscular rheumatism and arthritis.
Prepared as	Decoction, powder and tincture.

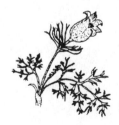

Pulsatilla

Prickly Ash
XANTHOXYLUM AMERICANUM

Also known as	Toothache tree
Where found	Canada and the United States
Appearance	Medium-sized tree
Parts used	Bark and berries
Therapeutic uses	The berries are carminative — they help ease griping pains in the stomach and intestinal tract, expel flatulence and reduce distension. Also helpful as a circulatory tonic and treatment for chronic rheumatism.
Prepared as	Decoction, fluid extract and tincture.

Pulsatilla
ANEMONE PULSATILLA

Also known as	Wind flower
Where found	Britain and Europe
Parts used	Leaves
Therapeutic uses	Sedative, nervine, antispasmodic. Helpful for women with menstrual problems and also for headaches associated with tension. Also indicated for insomnia and skin eruptions.
Prepared as	Infusion and tincture. Use only in small doses. Best used in combination with other remedies.

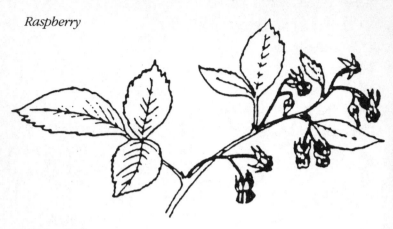

Raspberry
RUBUS IDAEUS

Where found	Common in gardens in most temperate climates
Appearance	A bush producing edible fruit
Part used	Leaves
Therapeutic uses	Astringent and stimulant. It is mild in action and soothing to the mucous lining of the stomach and intestinal tract. A useful remedy for simple diarrhoea in children. A gargle is used to soothe sore throats. The hormone-like action of raspberry tea explains its traditional use for easier and speedier labour in childbirth.
Prepared as	Infusion (which may be used as a gargle, lotion, and douche), tincture

Red Sage
SALVIA OFFICINALIS

Also known as	Garden sage
Where found	Commonly cultivated as a culinary herb in Europe and the United States
Appearance	A herb growing to about 12cm with purplish flowers
Part used	Leaves
Therapeutic uses	Good for those with poor digestion. It is an astringent with stimulating and carminative properties. Useful in dyspepsia and flatulence and in debilitated conditions. The infusion is also used as a gargle in sore throat, quinsy and laryngitis. It also helps prevent excessive perspiration. Contraindicated in pregnancy.
Prepared as	Infusion and tincture.

Rosemary
ROSMARINUS OFFICINALIS

Where found	A well known garden herb
Appearance	A shrubby herb with evergreen spiky leaves and small pale blue flowers.
part used	Leaves
Therapeutic uses	Drink an infusion of a few leaves to a cup of boiling water (infuse

for a few minutes only) if you have a headache caused by a stomach upset. It also eases flatulence and is an antifungal. Contraindicated in pregnancy.

Prepared as   Infusion.

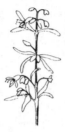

Rosemary

Senna
CASSIA ANGUSTIFOLIA

Where found	Egypt, Sudan, India.
Appearance	A shrub with greyish-green winged leaflets
Parts used	Leaves, pods.
Therapeutic uses	Laxative and cathartic. It is given only when it is necessary to clear the large intestine rapidly of faecal matter. It prevents straining to produce a stool which is important in those with hiatus hernia. It should be combined with aromatic herbs such as Cloves, Ginger, Cinnamon or Aniseed to prevent griping pains.

Prepared as	Decoction, infusion, syrup, fluid extract, tincture. Not recommended in inflammatory bowel conditions.

Senna

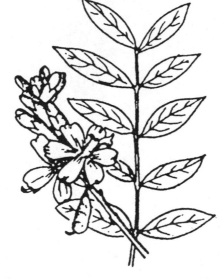

Stone Root
COLLINSONIA CANADENSIS

Also known as	Heal-all
Where found	Canada
Appearance	Woodland plant with large greenish-yellow flowers.
Part used	Root
Therapeutic uses	Gastrointestinal tonic and antispasmodic indicated in gastroenteritis and haemorrhoids.
Prepared as	Decoction and tincture.

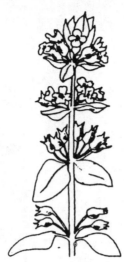

Thyme
THYMUS VULGARIS

Where found	Common garden plant.
Appearance	Small perennial herb with tiny leaves.
Part used	Herb.
Therapeutic uses	Antispasmodic and tonic. Contains thymol, a strong antiseptic, useful in irritable coughs and catarrh. People with hiatus hernia need chronic coughs to be treated to prevent unnecessary strain on the chest.
Prepared as	Infusion, sweetened with honey and given in tablespoonful doses. Not to be taken during pregnancy.

74

Valerian
VALERIAN OFFICINALIS

Also known as	All heal
Where found	Near streams, rivers and ditches in Britain.
Appearance	Grows to about a metre in height with pinkish white flowers.
Part used	Rhizome
Therapeutic uses	Nervine, sedative and antispasmodic. Combined with ginger for the treatment of abdominal colic and cramps, stomach pains and diarrhoea. Excellent for relieving nervous tension and debility. Promotes sleep.
Prepared as	Decoction, fluid extract and tincture.

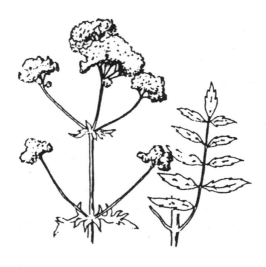

Valerian

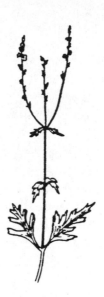

Vervain
VERBENA OFFICINALIS

Also known as	Herb of Grace
Where found	By roadsides and in meadows in Britain.
Appearance	A perennial trailing herb bearing small pale-lilac flowers.
Part used	Leaves
Therapeutic uses	It improves liver function and clears mucous from the stomach and intestinal canal. It is antispasmodic and a blood purifier. It is also an excellent nervine helping to lift depression and ease tension.

Wild Yam
DIOSCOREA VILLOSA

Also known as	Colic Root.
Where found	Tropical countries, United States and Canada.
Appearance	A perennial climbing plant.
Part used	Root
Therapeutic uses	Useful in hiatus hernia as it has a specific action on the pylorus, the lower sphincter muscle of the stomach. It is an antispasmodic and will relieve nausea, flatulence and colic. Also used in neuralgia, sickness in pregnancy, asthma, cramping pains, painful periods, uterine pain and rheumatism arising from liver and digestive disorders.
Prepared as	Decoction, fluid extract and tincture. Note: dried root quickly loses its therapeutic potency.

Witch Hazel
HAMAMELIS VIRGINIANA

Where found	United States and Canada
Appearance	Similar to an apple tree
Parts used	Bark and leaves
Therapeutic uses	An astringent indicated in hiatus hernia where there is bleeding from the bowel. It is also a

general tonic and sedative. Other uses: witch hazel is a popular remedy for painful, bleeding piles, particularly in cases where the bowels are loose.

Prepared as   Decoction, tincture, distilled water, ointment and suppositories.

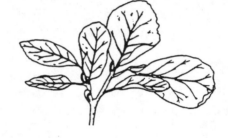

Witch Hazel

Wood Betony
BETONICA OFFICINALIS

Also known as	Bishopswort
Where found	Woodland in Europe
Appearance	A broad-leaved plant with spikes of red flowers spotted white.
Parts used	Leaves, or whole herb.
Therapeutic uses	A general tonic particularly useful in conditions where both nerves and stomach are involved, such as stomach pain and headaches due to digestive conditions. Helps alleviate dyspepsia.
Prepared as	Decoction, infusion and tincture.

Yarrow
ACHILLEA MILLEFOLIUM

Also known as	Nosebleed, Milfoil, Thousand-leaf
Where found	Roadsides, meadows and waste ground in Britain.
Appearance	An upright plant growing to about 61cm with leaves divided into a multitude of parts, hence the name thousand-leaf. The flowers are white or pink with yellowish centres.
Part used	Herb.
Therapeutic uses	Tones the digestive tract and improves the appetite. Especially useful where there is intestinal bleeding and where the bowels are loose. Also used for bleeding piles. The hot infusion induces sweating making it an excellent remedy in colds, flu and catarrh: combine with peppermint.
Prepared as	Cold infusion, hot infusion (for colds), tincture.

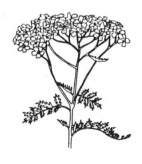

Yarrow

Chapter 14

The Comfrey Dilemma

There is no doubt that comfrey — known to country folk as knitbone, and for good reason — has for years been an excellent treatment for hiatus hernia and other diseases.

At present, however, herbalists face a dilemma in advocating its use due to research conducted in Australia which has put comfrey under a cloud.

The facts are that comfrey has a soothing and healing action on all injured, inflamed and ulcerated tissues. It is called knitbone because of its efficacy in healing broken bones faster than one would normally expect. Many cases of broken bones which have refused to heal have responded to treatment with comfrey.

The medical profession was cynical about the healing properties of comfrey until research showed that it contained a substance which encourages wound healing. The substance, allantoin, is now made synthetically for that purpose, and is also used in skin preparations.

In ulcerated conditions, as may accompany hiatus hernia, it stimulates the healing process by helping to form epithelium, the surface layer of the skin. It has been used for centuries for both internal ulceration, such as peptic and duodenal ulcer and for external ulcers, such as occur, for example, on the legs of people with poor circulation, or with blood diseases.

But using the plant is far superior to just using the isolated allantoin. Comfrey also contains copious amounts of mucilage which acts as an emollient, coating the tissues and preventing further damage. It also has astringent properties which work to check haemorrhage.

Culpepper, the English herbalist (1616-1654) was quite accurate when he said ... "The root boiled and the decoction drunk helps all inward hurts, bruises, wounds and ulcers. The roots outwardly applied help fresh wounds, or cuts, and are especially good for broken bones and ruptures."

The healing properties of comfrey root are at their best in early spring when all the goodness is stored there, and at their lowest in midsummer when all the virtues have been dispersed into the leaves. One can make a decoction from the leaves and use it for all the same purposes but it will not be so effective as the root.

For hiatus hernia comfrey has been used in combination with a decoction of slippery elm, another exceptional healing agent.

The dilemma over comfrey arises out of an Australian study which has revealed that pyrrozolidine alkaloids in the leaves and roots produced liver damage in rats.

The researchers concluded that comfrey could possibly cause cancer in humans and should be banned.

As far as I am aware there has never been a case of cancer reported in humans due to the use of comfrey.

On the contrary it has been reported, though not in recent times, that comfrey has been used successfully in the treatment of stomach cancer.

The problem for the researchers is that pyrrozolidine alkaloids are found naturally in many of our everyday foods, some of which contain higher amounts than in comfrey.

Comfrey is also a plant that horses and other herbivorous animals nibble when they are grazing. They usually know what is good for them and what is not. As a result comfrey has been incorporated for years into animal feed, presumably without any obvious detrimental effects. But is it a food that rats naturally consume?

Organic gardeners have used comfrey leaves in the production of compost for their vegetable gardens. The observation to date surely is that people who consume organic produce are much less likely to suffer ill health than those who consume processed foods.

At the time of writing there have been no moves in the UK by the Department of Health or by the Medicines Control Agency to recommend the cessation of the internal use of comfrey as a herbal medicine. Comfrey tablets are produced by leading herbal manufacturers and are still available at health food shops. There is also no problem with the use of comfrey externally in the form of powder, infused oil, ointment or poultice.

I have included this information about comfrey because it is possible that the situation could change as a result of further research. In any event there are moves among horticulturists to try to produce comfrey with low, or no, levels of pyrrozolidine alkaloids. In the meantime, my advice is to reserve the use of comfrey to that of an external healing agent.

Chapter 15

Exercise —
Helpful or Harmful?

Breathing exercises to improve the tone of the diaphragm and gentle exercises to tone up muscles are an important part of naturopathic treatment.

An overall general exercise programme which includes walking, jogging, swimming, or yoga is the best way to start.

Vigorous exercise is not advocated as sudden exaggerated movements may trigger hiatus hernia in the unfit.

Exercises which put a strain on the abdomen, like lying on the floor with the legs straight and then raising both legs up together, or hanging from a beam and raising the legs, should be avoided.

Strenuous sports like squash and weight-lifting, can be an associated factor in hiatus hernia, and are best left to the younger set.

Concentrate on breathing properly while out walking or jogging.

LIFTING

Lifting and carrying heavy weights can trigger off the symptoms of hiatus hernia and may aggravate the condition where it is already established.

But when lifting is unavoidable one should always remember to lift a heavy object by using the power of the thigh muscles. Bend the knees and keep the back straight, do not bend over from the waist with the legs straight as this puts a strain on to the abdominal muscles.

Chapter 16

Seeking Professional Help

Although this book is aimed at giving those with hiatus hernia syndrome information and guidance on the herbal and naturopathic approach to treatment, it cannot be stressed too much that quicker results can often be achieved by consulting a fully qualified herbal or naturopathic practitioner.

When treatment is being conducted by a medical herbalist the functioning of the whole body will be taken into account and, therefore, the prescription will vary from one individual to another.

There may be internal haemorrhage which requires attention. Herbal medicines may also be required to be taken for co-existing conditions, such as an ulcer or gallstones.

Patients are seen by appointment and in confidence in the practitioner's consulting rooms. Herbal practitioners qualified with the National Institute of Medical Herbalists, can be recognised by the initials MNIMH or FNIMH after their names. They are trained to deal with a wide range of medical problems, although some practitioners may specialise in certain medical areas.

Naturopaths trained at the British College of Naturopathy and Osteopathy in London and admitted to the Register of Naturopaths have the letters ND MRN after their names.

They are specialists in the non-drug treatment of a wide variety of conditions, although many naturopaths specialise in musculoskeletal problems.

The National Institute of Medical Herbalists, founded in 1864, is the oldest established body of practising medical herbalists in the world. Members can be found in most towns in the UK. The easiest way to find out if there is one near you is to look under 'Herbalists' in Yellow Pages, Thomson's, or other local directory.

The aim of both naturopathy and herbal medicine is not just to relieve symptoms but to offer the sufferer an increased level of general health. The practitioner takes an holistic approach to his patients, an approach that is being followed more and more by other primary health care practitioners.

He will, therefore, take into account not only the physical symptoms of hiatus hernia but also any mental stress or emotional problems which may be relevant.

Both the body and the mind conform to the laws of nature, one of the most important of which is the law of homoeostasis — the ability of the individual to be self-regulating, despite changes in the environment.

It is the law of balance that has enabled us to survive for thousands of years despite changes, or threats, in the environment, whether it be a simple change in temperature, or an infection due to pathogenic micro-organisms.

Disease is produced when outside threats, or changes, are too overwhelming and the individual fails to respond or adapt healthily.

It is not always easy to treat oneself appropriately. It quite often needs a trained practitioner to give guidance so that the deeper reasons for an illness and not just the superficial are treated.

Glossary of Common Medical Terms

Very often when reading, or on having a medical consultation, words are used which may not be familiar. This short list will help to make some of the more common ones a little clearer.

Alterative
A medicine that beneficially alters the process of nutrition and restores the normal function of an organ or bodily system. In herbal medicine it usually refers to a remedy that purifies the blood by improving the function of the organs, such as liver and kidneys, which are involved in this process.

Amenorrhoea
Absence of menstrual periods during the years when they should normally be present.

Analgesic
A medicine that blocks or relieves pain.

Anodyne
A medicine that alleviates pain — physical or mental.

Anthelmintic
A medicine that is used to rid the body of intestinal worms.

Antiphlogistic   A medicine, or agent, which reduces inflammation or fever.

Antipyretic   A medicine, or method, used to lower the body temperature to normal. In naturopathic medicine, cold baths, and spongeing or application of ice packs are used to combat fever.

Antiseptic   A medicine, or other substance, that prevents putrefaction.

Antispasmodic   A remedy that prevents or relieves colic or spasms. Among the most potent antispasmodics derived from plants are belladonna and opium. Naturopathic antispasm is achieved with the application of hot compresses and fomentations.

Aperient   A remedy that produces a natural movement of the bowels.

Aphrodisiac   A substance that is reputed to produce sexual desire and stimulate the sexual organs.

Astringent   Binding or contracting tissues.

Cardiac   Relating to the heart, either a medicine, or disease, that alters heart function.

Carminative   A medicine that eases griping pains and flatulence in the bowel.

Cathartic   A strong laxative, or purgative, producing evacuation of the bowels.

Corrective   Correcting or counteracting the harmful and restoring to a healthy state.

Debility	Feebleness of health; run down.
Degenerative	A disease that results in destruction or disintegration of tissue.
Demulcent	A soothing medicine, mostly applied to those that act on the gastrointestinal canal.
Deobstruent	Removing obstructions and opening the ducts and other natural passages of the body.
Diaphoretic	A substance that induces perspiration.
Diuretic	A substance that increases the flow of urine.
Dysmenorrhoea	Excessive pain during menstruation
Dyspnoea	Breathlessness
Emetic	Any substance that causes vomiting.
Emmenagogue	A remedy that brings on the menstrual period.
Emollient	A medicine that softens, soothes and lubricates skin and internal tissues.
Haematemesis	Vomiting blood
Haemoptysis	Coughing up of blood
Haemostatic	A substance that checks bleeding and aids clotting of the blood.
Insecticide	Any substance fatal to insects.
Laxative	A substance that induces gentle, and easy bowel movement.
Leucorrhoea	A mucous discharge from the female genital organs, previously known as "the whites".

Menorrhagia   Excessive flow of menstrual blood.

Myalgia   Muscular pain; muscular rheumatism.

Narcotic   A drug that produces drowsiness, sleep, stupor and insensibility.

Nephritic   Relating to the kidneys.

Nervine   A remedy that relieves a nerve disorder and restores the nervous system to its normal state.

Oxytocic   A drug that causes contractions of the uterus and hastens childbirth.

Parturient   A remedy used during childbirth.

Purgative   A medicine taken to evacuate the bowels, but one that is much stronger than a laxative or aperient.

Resolvent   A drug, application, or other substance that reduces swellings and tumours.

Rubefacient   A treatment that produces redness, inflammation and blisters of the skin; a counter-irritant (rubefy = make red).

Sedative   A remedy soothing to the nervous system; a tranquilliser.

Soporific   Promoting sleep.

Stimulant   A remedy that produces a rapid increase in vital energy of part or of the whole body.

Stomachic   Relating to the stomach; a remedy that aids the normal function of the stomach, promoting proper digestion and appetite.

Stricture	The narrowing of any of the natural passages of the body, such as the urethra, the bowel or the gullet.
Styptic	A substance that checks bleeding.
Sudorific	A remedy that produces heavy perspiration.
Tonic	A medicine that invigorates or tones up a part or the whole of the body and promotes wellbeing.
Vermifuge	A medicine that expels worms from the body.
Vulnerary	An ointment or treatment that promotes the healing of wounds.

Your Story

If you have benefited from using herbal medicine, for hiatus hernia syndrome or any allied condition, either from home use or from those prescribed by professional medical herbalists or naturopaths, you are invited to send details to the author of this series of books, c/o the publishers, W. Foulsham & Co. Ltd, Yeovil Road, Slough, Berkshire SL1 4JH. Unfortunately, the author regrets that he is unable to enter into any correspondence on this matter.

FURTHER READING

Other books in this series include:

Skin Problems
Arthritis and Rheumatism
Stress and Nervous Tension
Sexual Problems
Irritable Bowel Syndrome

The Author

David Potterton is one of a few practitioners in Britain who are qualified in both herbal and naturopathic medicine.

A member of the National Institute of Medical Herbalists (NIMH) and of the British Naturopathic Association (BNA), he is also member of the General Council and Register of Naturopaths.

Mr Potterton has been a member of the McCarrison Society — a medical organisation devoted to the study of health and nutrition — for several years.

He was also a member of the Royal Society of Medicine for many years and a member of the Vegetarian Society's research committee.

Mr Potterton has been tutor in materia medica and in pathology for the NIMH, and has conducted a series of further education lecture courses on herbal medicine. He also lectures frequently to local organisations and health workers.

As a writer, Mr Potterton has contributed to all the major health magazines in the UK, including "Here's Health" and "Healthy Living", and was the English editor of "Bestways", the American health magazine.

He was medical editor of the family doctor newspaper "Doctor" for many years, and co-editor of the "British Journal of Phytotherapy", a professional journal for herbal practitioners and naturopathic physicians.

He is the editor of several books published by Foulsham, including "Culpeper's Colour Herbal" and "Medicinal Plants".

He has also revised and edited a number of Foulsham books on herbal medicine in this series, including "Arthritis and Rheumatism", "Skin Problems", "Stress and Tension" and "Sexual Problems". He is also the author of "Irritable Bowel Syndrome", published by Foulsham.